Detox Tea: The Ultimate Guide to Detoxifying your Body with Healthy Homemade Tea

Disclaimer and Terms of Use: Effort has been made to ensure that the information in this book is accurate and complete, however, the author and the publisher do not warrant the accuracy of the information, text and graphics contained within the book due to the rapidly changing nature of science, research, known and unknown facts and internet. The Author and the publisher do not hold any responsibility for errors, omissions or contrary interpretation of the subject matter herein. This book is presented solely for motivational and informational purposes only.

Table of Contents

Southern Sweet Tea

Ingredients:
- 3 C water
- 2 Family tea bags
- ¾ C Sugar
- 7 C cold ice water

Directions:

I. Bring 3 C water to a boil and add the tea bags for 1 minute then remove from heat and cover and set
II. Throw bags away and add your sugar, until sugar dissolves
III. Pour into container and add the ice cold water
IV. Serve with ice

Lemon Berry Sweet Tea

Ingredients:
- 1 pkg frozen blueberries
- ½ C fresh lemon juice
- 3 family size tea bags
- ¾ C sugar

Directions:

I. Boil blueberries and lemon juice stirring often
II. Remove from heat and add 4 C water, bring to a boil adding 3 tea bags, once boiling get rid of bags and add sugar an blue berry mixture
III. Pour into pitcher, chill and serve

Sweet Tea Tiramisu

Ingredients:

- 2 tea bags
- 2 containers mascarpone cheese
- 1 T vanilla extract
- 2 C whipping cream
- 1 pkgs lady fingers
- 2 T unsweetened cocoa

Directions:

I. Boil 4 C water and add tea bags, remove from heat and let sit. Remove tea bags

II. Add sugar and stir until dissolve. Let boil 20-22 minutes Let cool

III. Stir in cheese and vanilla extract, and ½ C sugar

IV. Beat whipping cream until stiff and fold into cheese

V. Arrange halved ladyfingers in baking dish and pour tea batter over it and drop with cheese mixture, then repeat. Sift cocoa over it then serve

Blackberry Sweet Tea

Ingredients:
- 2 C frozen blackberries
- 1 ¼ C sugar
- 1 T fresh mint
- Baking soda
- 4 C boiling water
- 2 family size tea bags
- 2 ½ C cold water

Directions:

I.   Blend your blackberries and sugar and crush
II.   Stir in mint and baking soda
III.   Pour boiling water over tea bags and steep. Throw away tea bags
IV.   Pour tea over blackberries and let sit at room temperature, strain and add cold water stirring until sugar dissolves.
V.   Chill for 1-2 hours and serve

Christmas Tea

Ingredients:
- 1 gal. unsweetened tea
- 1 can pineapple juice
- ½ gallon lemonade
- ½ gallon orange juice
- ½ gallon cranberry juice
- ½ gallon apple juice
- 2 C sugar
- 1 pkg. mulling spices
- 1 bottle ginger ale

Directions:

I.   Stir everything together in a 5 gallon pitcher and chill for a few hours. Stir in ginger ale right before serving

Apple Pomegranate Cider

Ingredients:
- Cloves
- Cinnamon sticks
- Lemon rind
- 8 C apple cider
- 1 C pomegranate juice
- ¾ C orange juice
- ¼ C sugar
- ¼ C lemon juice

Directions:

I.   Add first four ingredients in a cheese cloth bag and dunk in mixture of other ingredient, bringing to a boil,

II.   Throw away cheesecloth bag

III.   Serve

Age Defy Tea

Ingredients:
- 1 ginger root
- 1 tsp Turmeric
- 1 T fresh mint
- 1 C purified water

Directions:

I.   Boil your water and pour over ingredients, strain
II.   Serve

Metabolism Booster

Ingredients:
- 2 chopped garlic cloves
- 1 tsp cayenne pepper
- 1 C water

Directions:

I.   Boil water and pour over the cayenne pepper stir in garlic and serve

Morning Detox tea

Ingredients:
- 1 C green tea
- 1 slice lemon
- 1 tsp raw honey

Directions:

I. Boil water with the tea bag, boil for 3-4 minutes
II. Remove bag, pour tea over lemon and honey
III. Serve

Fat Burning Tea

Ingredients:
- 1 tsp cinnamon
- 1 lemon wedge
- 1 C water

Directions:

I.   Boil your water and add the cinnamon, stirring in cinnamon and squeezing lemon juice into cinnamon water

II.   Serve

Cancer Shield Tea

Ingredients:
- ½ C Dandelion tea
- ½ C chamomile tea

Directions:

I.   Combine these two prepared cups of tea and enjoy

Hang over Detox tea

Ingredients:
- 1 C milk thistle tea
- 1 tsp coconut milk

Directions:

I.   Pour brewed tea into bug with coconut milk and serve

Reset Detox Tea

Ingredients:
- ½ tsp peppermint
- ½ tsp alfalfa
- ½ tsp stinging Nettle
- ½ tsp Eucalyptus
- 1 C water

Directions:

I. Chop your leaves and boil water and add leaves,
II. Strain brewed tea and serve

Jillian Michaels Tea

Ingredients:
- 6 oz. water
- 2 T lemon juice
- 1 T sugar free cranberry Juice
- 1 dandelion root tea bag

Directions:

I.   Boil water and brew tea,
II.   Pour brewed tea over cranberry juice and lemon

Belly Shrinker Tea

Ingredient:
- 3 slices cucumber
- Lemon
- ½ T ginger
- Mint leaves
- ½ T honey

Directions:

I.   Slice your cucumber and squeeze lemon juice into water
II.   Grate or ground your ginger and add to water
III. Add mint, and honey and stir
IV.   Serve

Green Tea

Ingredients:
- 1 C green tea, brewed
- ½ C baby Kale
- ½ apple, cored
- 1 T Greek Yogurt
- Ice

Directions:

I.   Add everything into your blender and blend. You may add avocado for added texture if you prefer

Fruity Green Tea

Ingredients:

- 1 C brewed green tea
- ½ pear, sliced
- ½ C pineapple
- ½ C papaya, sliced

Directions:

I.   Cube or slice all of your fruits and add to your blender or juicer. You want this to be juicy

II.   You want no texture.

III.   Serve

Good morning Green Tea

Ingredients:
- 1 tsp Green tea Match powder
- ½ Orange, sliced
- ¼ grapefruit, sliced
- ½ banana
- 1 C coconut milk
- Ice

Directions:

I.   Blend everything until thick like a milkshake

Tea Frappe

Ingredients:
- 1 tsp green tea patch powder
- 1 C coconut milk
- Ice

Directions:

I.   Blend and serve

Tropical Green Tea Shake

Ingredients:
- 1 tsp green tea match powder
- ½ fresh mango
- ½ C papaya, cubed
- ½ banana
- 1 C coconut milk
- Ice

Directions:

I.   Blend and serve

Spiced Tonic

Ingredients:
- 1 C brewed and chilled Green tea
- ¼ C blueberries
- ¼ C raspberries
- 1 T Greek Yogurt
- Ice

Directions:

I.   Blend until smooth and serve

Mint Iced Green Tea

Ingredients:
- 1 C Fresh mint leaves
- 3 tea bags
- Ice
- Honey

Directions

I.   Add mint to bottom of pitcher and add tea bags, add boiling water and refrigerate for up to 6 hours, no less than 4 hours.
II. Add honey and serve

Skin detoxed

Ingredients:
- Green tea
- Agave
- Apple cider vinegar

Directions:

I.   Blend everything together and serve

Green Tea Lemonade

Ingredients:
- 1 bag green tea
- 2 T sugar
- ½ C boiling water
- 2 lemons juiced
- 8 oz. cold water
- Ice
- Lemon wedges to garnish

Directions:

I.   Add tea bag to boiling water and take off heat. Let sit for 3-5 minutes

II.   Stir in lemon juices

III. Pour into glass and serve

www.ingramcontent.com/pod-product-compliance
Lightning Source LLC
Chambersburg PA
CBHW071347310526
45790CB00018B/1386